W9-ARN-289

*Welcome to your Walking Stick Press guided
journal. Within these pages you'll find:*

*

instruction to guide you on your way

*

writing prompts to lead you to your goal

*

blank pages to record your responses to the
prompts—to map your insights as you heal, grow,
and explore

*

quotations to inspire, provoke, and refresh you

*

*Along the way, feel free to jot in the margins,
add your own quotes,
let writing take you down a trail you didn't expect.
Enjoy the journey.*

*

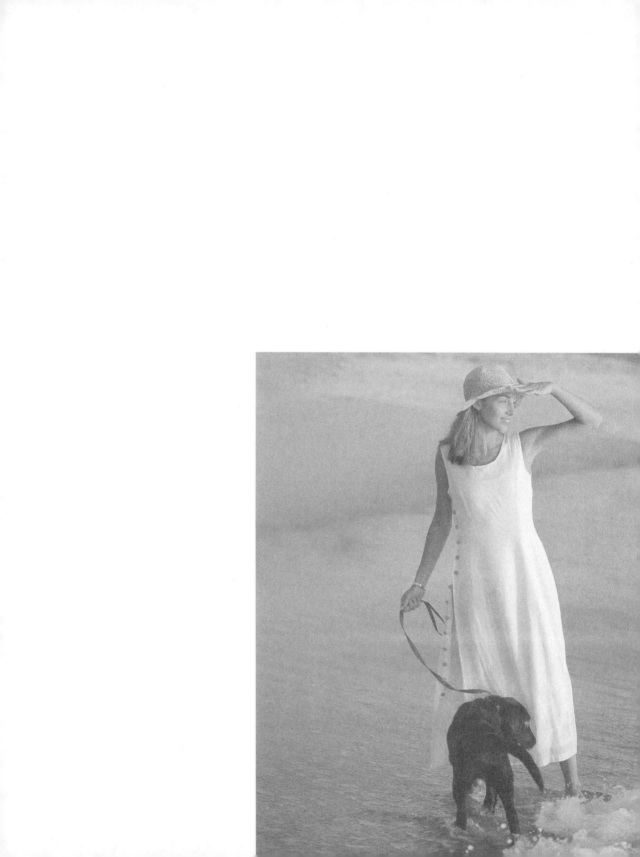

Body Confident

A Guided Journal for Losing Weight and Feeling Great

Victoria Moran

Walking Stick Press
Cincinnati, Ohio
www.writersdigest.com

Body Confident. Copyright © 2002 by Victoria Moran. Manufactured in the United States of America. All rights reserved. No part of this book may be reproduced in any form or by any electronic or mechanical means including information storage and retrieval systems without permission in writing from the publisher, except by a reviewer, who may quote brief passages in a review. Published by Walking Stick Press, an imprint of F&W Publications, Inc., 1507 Dana Avenue, Cincinnati, Ohio 45207. (800) 289-0963. First edition.

Visit our Web site at www.writersdigest.com for information on more resources for writers.

To receive a free weekly E-mail newsletter delivering tips and updates about writing and about Writer's Digest products, send an E-mail with "Subscribe Newsletter" in the body of the message to newsletter-request@writersdigest.com, or register directly at our Web site at www.writersdigest.com.

06 05 04 03 02   5 4 3 2 1

Library of Congress Cataloging-in-Publication Data

Moran, Victoria.
   Body confident: a guided journal for losing weight and feeling great / by Victoria Moran.
     p. cm.
   Includes bibliographical references.
   ISBN 1-58297-100-5
1. Weight loss. 2. Diaries--Authorship. I. Title.

RM222.2.M5675 2002
613.7-dc21   2001046521

Edited by Donya Dickerson and Meg Leder
Cover designed by Joanna Detz
Interior designed by Brian Roeth
Page layout by Donna Cozatchy
Cover photography by John Chillingworth/Hulton Archive
Production coordinated by Kristen Heller

dedication

To you, the reader and co-writer of this book:
May you come to know yourself better
and appreciate yourself more.

about the author

Victoria Moran has been called a "wellness visionary," and yet her work grew out of finding answers to her own struggle with food and weight. Her other books include:

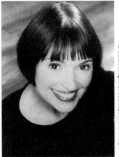

Credit: Joseph Orecchio, Studio Max, NYC

* *My Yoga Journal: Guided Reflections Through Writing,* another in this series of guided journals.
* *Lit from Within: Tending Your Soul for Lifelong Beauty.*
* *Creating a Charmed Life: Sensible, Spiritual Secrets Every Busy Woman Should Know.*
* *Shelter for the Spirit: How to Make Your Home a Haven in a Hectic World.*
* *Love Yourself Thin: The Revolutionary Spiritual Approach to Weight Loss.*

Moran's articles have appeared in publications including *Ladies' Home Journal, Woman's Day, Personal Journaling,* and *Yoga Journal.* She also speaks to businesses, associations, and churches around the country about how to make life richer, fuller, and healthier. For more information about her work or to invite Victoria Moran to speak to your organization, visit her Web site, www.victoriamoran.com.

table of **contents**

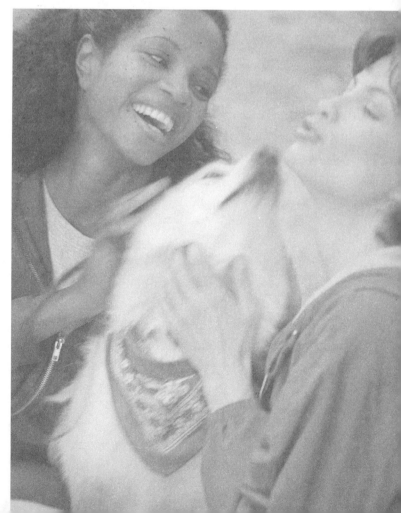

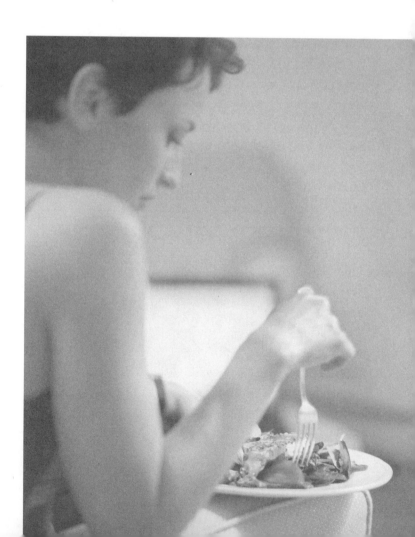

introduction

You've probably heard the axiom, "If you do what you've always done, you'll get what you always got." Congratulations! You're about to do something different about losing weight, getting fit, and feeling better about the shape you're in.

In purchasing this journal in which to record your food and your feelings, you have set yourself apart from the typical person who wants to lose weight. You have decided to stop battling your body and instead learn more about the person who inhabits it. The result will be a vastly improved relationship with food, your body, and yourself.

In my own case, freedom from an obsession with food and weight started when I gave up the fight. I had dieted nearly all my life. My parents were both in the weight-loss business—my father as a physician, my mom as the manager of "reducing salons," the precursor to health clubs but characterized by lavender carpeting and "passive exercise machines." I grew up knowing two ways to eat: the diet and the binge. Eventually, I lost the ability to diet at will, and whether I was wearing my "fat clothes" or my "thin clothes" that week, I invariably felt out of control.

In this defeated state, I realized I had gone on my last

diet. I had to become willing to live at peace with the body I had, while trying to eat as reasonably as I was able and exercise as sanely as I could. That meant that I'd eat more and exercise less than when I'd dieted, and eat less and exercise more than when I'd stuffed myself in front of the TV. In other words, I aimed to become *balanced* in this part of my life in which I'd formerly been anything but.

I started slowly, tentatively. And I cushioned myself with support: a group of other people who also wanted to eat sensibly and live well; a health club where looking like the cover girl of the *Sports Illustrated* swimsuit issue was not the goal; and a spiral-bound journal I labeled simply "Musings." I figured I'd read enough diet books to last a lifetime. I was ready to write one—not for public consumption, but for me.

Those initial musings introduced me to the art and science of keeping a journal as a companion and guide during the weight-loss process and beyond. I wrote what I ate, and even more importantly I wrote what I felt, what bothered me, what delighted me, and what I learned.

With *Body Confident*, you can learn more about yourself, too. This is *your* book. What I've written offers information and inspiration for you, but what you write is the key to your transformation. You have your own wisdom about food, exercise, the way you look, the way you want to look, the way you live, and the way you want to live. Writing gives you access to this wisdom.

Most of the blank pages in this volume are for free writing or "life journaling." This is a revealing process. You may find that the problems you've had with weight are less a matter of what you're eating than what's been eating you. You can use this journal in ways that serve you best. For example:

* **You can write to get a clear view of your current lifestyle.** Through writing about the kinds of foods you

like, the way you cook, the restaurants you frequent, and the exercise you do (or don't do), you can get an accurate picture of what's going right and what isn't.

* **You can work through problems (with food and other things, too) by writing about them.** Writing can defuse anger and frustration; it can also help you come up with viable solutions to many of life's inevitable predicaments.

* **You may wish to explore the mind-sets that have stood in your way in the past.** Deep-seated attitudes and issues are at the root of some people's excessive eating or unhealthful food choices. Although keeping a journal is not a substitute for therapy, it is a therapeutic tool that can lead you to a great many "aha!" moments—revelations about yourself you'll be glad you've had.

A list of writing prompts precedes each group of blank pages. These are questions to answer and ideas to ponder on paper. Some are playful, almost like games, but all are designed to facilitate your progress. You don't need to respond to every prompt; choose the ones that jump out at you. And allow your writing to take you where it wants to go.

Let this be a journey of self-discovery. For example, you may respond to a prompt dealing with exercise by writing about the difficulty you've had lately in getting to step class or aqua-aerobics on time. This thought may lead you to expound upon tardiness in general. Don't think you need to steer yourself back to the topic of exercise. You need to be writing about what you're writing about or you wouldn't be doing it. Trust yourself here.

In addition to the free writing pages, you'll also find *Nourish & Nurture* boxes in which to record (1) what you eat each day, (2) the exercise you do (if this is an exercise day for

nourish
and nurture

Food I ate today:

B—Poached egg, rye toast, 6oz. o.j., decaf coffee/skim milk—took multi-vitamin and extra C

L—Caesar salad, hard roll, shared creme brulee with Jennifer, iced tea

3 o'clock—Persimmon—never had one before—really good

D—Chicken-veggie stir-fry over rice, steamed broccoli, lemon sorbet, herbal (chamomile) tea.

Exercise I did:

Formal: gym—weight training 40 mins.
Other: Walked from car to office (8 bl. total)
Walked dog (30 mins.)

Something to care for me:

Took long bath with candles—shut off phone

you), and (3) something you did to nurture yourself, to treat yourself especially well.

Write down what you eat whether it's perfect (whatever that is), so-so, or not so hot. You aren't being graded. An important function of keeping a food journal is to obtain information. What do you eat when you're left to your own devices? How could you realistically do it better? What circumstances make it hard for you to eat in a reasonable way? Can some of these circumstances be avoided or at least better prepared for?

In the space marked for exercise in the *Nourish & Nurture* boxes, write the activity you did and a few words about how it felt. "Ran in the park—20 minutes—more stamina than yesterday," or "Aerobics class—1 hour—kept wishing I looked better in spandex." On the days you've scheduled for not working out, write something positive in the exercise space. "Holiday!" works for me.

The nurture section may seem superfluous, but that's because we live in a culture that has an overinflated work ethic. We feel guilty when we get the pleasure we want. To become body confident, however, nurturing yourself is essential. To an unnurtured person, the refrigerator and the couch look awfully good. Minimize their lure by indulging yourself in a manicure, a long conversation with a special friend, or by taking your full lunch hour for a change and relaxing at a pleasant café.

Soon journal-keeping itself will become a nurturing activity for you. And when you finish this journal, you'll possess the travelog of a private journey, a diary of self-knowledge and personal growth.

Oftentimes people think of a weight-loss program in terms of what they're giving up. Some even have a "last meal" the night before as if they're going to be executed at daybreak. With the help of *Body Confident,* your experience will be different. The ideas presented in this book do not describe a process of deprivation but of *exploration* in which reaching a number on a scale becomes secondary to growing confident about the way you look and enthusiastic about the way you live. With this new state of mind, you will shed pounds, and more importantly, they won't come looking for you later.

check in

At the end of each chapter, you'll find a Check In page. Whether you go through each chapter in a week, in a month, or at your own pace, use this page to help you focus on where you are in the process of achieving body confidence. What are your frustrations? What are your achievements?

Sample:

At the gym, I haven't been getting on the scale. That's progress.

I went to my sister's wedding and honestly didn't think about my body. I just had a good time.

I ate too much today. I was busy and got flustered. The good thing is, it's history. I don't have to go on eating this way.

what do i want from this book?

Describe what you think it means to be body confident. As you think of your definition, consider what steps you need to take to become more body confident and how you want to use this book to help you achieve your goals.

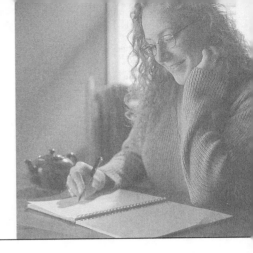

laying a healthy foundation

If you intend to take off weight and keep it off for life, you are planning to accomplish something at which 95 percent of people fail. The odds are dismal, but if you follow the path of the 5 percent who succeed instead of the 95 percent who don't, the odds are in your favor. Those who make it have a different *attitude,* a greater *willingness,* and a more sincere *commitment* than those who don't. With these principles in place, you can join the winners, no matter how many times you may have been disappointed before.

Attitude. Attitude is what you believe about yourself and your chances for success. The old way of thinking about weight loss—the way that didn't work—was to start with the premise, "I am a mess. If I don't lose this weight, I will never look good. I won't get promotions at work. My spouse will get tired of me." This outlook takes your energy away instead of giving you the extra energy you need for taking a brisk walk before lunch or for getting up early on Saturday to go to the farmers' market.

Instead, energize yourself with inner dialog like this: "I am an intelligent, attractive person with a great deal to give and to live for. I want to take better care of myself than I ever have so I can enjoy life even more and fulfill my potential."

If you're thinking that this motto sounds good but that the previous message (the one about being a mess) is closer to the truth, understand that although you may be overweight, even obese, you were designed to live in a healthy, attractive body. This is your birthright. It is the truth about you and it doesn't change. Circumstances—i.e., the shape your body is in—change all the time. You are, in fact, starting on a course to change them for the better right now as you read—and write—this book.

Willingness. When you're willing, you do what needs to be done, when you feel like it and when you don't. It takes a little extra effort. You may need to rearrange your schedule a few days a week to fit in exercise. Or change classroom volunteer jobs with another parent: You can drive for field trips; for now, let her bake the cookies.

Willingness also implies flexibility. The diet mentality is rigid: "This is what you eat, no matter what." But life isn't like that. In real life, there are holidays and foods that go with them. There are Sunday brunches, business lunches, day trips to the country and dream trips to Paris. You need to be willing to keep your eating within prudent boundaries but still be flexible enough to be part of all this *living*.

Commitment. No one who loses weight and keeps it off does so without a sincere commitment to a new way of life. The particulars are up to you. The commitment is to refuse to go back to where you came from.

You will not eat an absolutely flawless diet every day for the rest of your life. What is crucial is that you allow for less than exemplary days and stay on your path anyway. When you are committed to becoming body confident, you don't let inevitable ups and downs impede your progress. You're worth going the distance.

writing prompts

Let these suggestions spur your writing.
Don't feel the need to respond to all of them;
just write about the ones that speak to your heart.

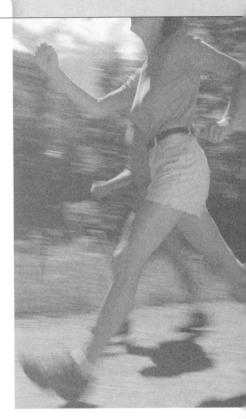

1. How do you feel about your physical self? Write what you like about it, what you don't, and how writing about it makes you feel. Let the words flow.

2. Write a letter to your body. If you feel you owe it an apology for not treating it as well as it deserves or for thinking ill of it, do that. Ask your body to let you know what it needs—nutritionally and every other way. The body can be really good at this. Pregnant women's cravings for foods that contain nutrients they're missing are a case in point.

3. Write another letter, this one a letter of recommendation for yourself as if it were for someone else—not to help them get a better job, but to live a richer life. Make this a glowing recommendation. Write it in the third person and be specific, not just "Jane is nice," but "Friends turn to Jane for help first because they know she'll come through for them."

4. Draw up a time line of your past experiences losing weight—the dates, the diets, the outcomes. Then get the disappointment of those efforts that didn't last down on paper. End the time line with the present, and discuss how you're doing things in a new way.

5. Make a list of what you are willing to do today to help yourself be healthier and happier. Then pick one entry from your list and resolve to do that one thing today. Write tomorrow about how your efforts went.

how is my foundation?

Take some time to consider the three personality traits brought up in this section. Describe your current *attitude, commitment,* and *willingness* about losing weight. Then, every few weeks, reflect on what you've written to see if your foundation is still in place.

Attitude

Commitment

Willingness

nourish
and nurture

Food I ate today:

Exercise I did:

Something to care for me:

nourish
and nurture

Food I ate today:

Exercise I did:

Something to care for me:

*I believe one writes because
one has to create a world in
which one can live.*

ANAÏS NIN

nourish *and nurture*

Food I ate today:

Exercise I did:

Something to care for me:

*Try to view self-doubt as
nothing more than a hiccup;
a simple reminder that you're
pushing yourself and
expanding your potential by
doing so.*

KRISTINE CARLSON,
*DON'T SWEAT THE SMALL
STUFF FOR WOMEN*

nourish *and nurture*

Food I ate today:

Exercise I did:

Something to care for me:

*Life is a banquet, and most
poor suckers are starving to
death.*

AUNTIE MAME

nourish
and nurture

Food I ate today:

Exercise I did:

Something to care for me:

nourish
and nurture

Food I ate today:

Exercise I did:

Something to care for me:

nourish *and nurture*

Food I ate today:

Exercise I did:

Something to care for me:

nourish
and nurture

Food I ate today:

Exercise I did:

Something to care for me:

It is never too late to be what you might have been.

GEORGE ELIOT

nourish
and nurture

Food I ate today:

Exercise I did:

Something to care for me:

Every night at bedtime, say this prayer: God, help me to accept the truth about myself, no matter how magnificent it is.

RHONDA HULL, PH.D.

*If we women honor and
cherish our physical bodies,
we can be in our own power.
Devaluing ourselves for not
being thin or not mirroring
society's standards of how our
physical body should look can
silence our creative voices.*

GAIL MCMEEKIN, *THE 12
SECRETS OF HIGHLY CREATIVE
WOMEN: A PORTABLE MENTOR*

nourish
and nurture

Food I ate today:

Exercise I did:

Something to care for me:

check in

Use this page to help you focus on where you are in the process of achieving body confidence. What are your frustrations? What are your achievements?

eating healthy food

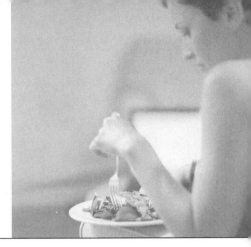

People used to think that losing weight meant eating very little and suffering quite a bit. Becoming body confident means eating in the healthiest way you know and making healthy foods delicious.

Nutrition is still a young science. Anyone who believed that the macronutrients (carbohydrates, protein, fat) and the micronutrients (vitamins and minerals) told the whole story got a surprise a few years back. That's when researchers began touting the wonders of *phytochemicals*—components of fruits, vegetables, beans, and even tea that are believed to help prevent a host of degenerative diseases, including many forms of cancer.

Because new findings about nutrition make their way into the media almost daily, anyone who wants to lose weight and eat more healthfully needs to both keep informed and stay steady. Otherwise, you'll be bouncing from one way of eating to another without ever finding something you'll stick with long enough to feel comfortable, safe, and grounded.

Once you have a basic plan for eating that makes sense to you (and to your physician if you're under a doctor's care), give it a chance. See how well it suits your physiology, your temperament, your family life. For most people, this is a way of eating that allows for dining out, entertaining, traveling, and the many other experiences that comprise a full life. Diets that are nutritionally marginal always backfire. And a rigid diet, whether it's nutritionally balanced or not, usually doesn't work because as much as we want to lose weight, we'd really rather live our lives.

The secret is to eat normally and moderately—the way someone who is already at your desired weight would eat. If you want to weigh 135 pounds and you now weigh 160, you are currently consuming enough calories to maintain a 160-pound body. If, instead, you eat enough calories to maintain a 135-pound body, you will eventually reach that weight. This means cutting back some and making wiser choices, but not depriving your body of the food it needs. The body's dual response to deprivation is: "Eat more as soon as you can get it," and "Store every calorie you can as fat; we'll need plenty on hand for the next famine."

Besides, any diet is by definition temporary. Instead, you need to adopt habits you can live with indefinitely. If you have a medical condition, it is imperative that you follow the instructions of your physician and dietician. Otherwise, carefully navigate through the maze of conflicting opinions about the right way to eat. There is a lot of misinformation out there, so weigh what you read and hear about diets against your own knowledge and your "gut feelings." Here are some points on which there is general agreement:

* **Eat enough so you're not hungry.** Hunger makes you think of one thing: food.

* **Avoid junk food on all but rare occasions.** Steer clear of gooey sweets, salty snacks, and deep-fried foods not so much because they're "bad" or "fattening" as because you deserve better. You are a quality human being who

deserves to eat quality food.

* **Stay away from any food that, instead of leaving you satisfied, causes you to want more of it.** Refined sugar products are the most common culprit, but sometimes white flour, peanut butter, cheese, or something else is a "binge food" for a particular individual. Respect your uniqueness. People who break out when they eat strawberries don't eat strawberries. Alcoholics who want their lives back don't drink alcohol. If eating sugar makes you hungrier than before you ate it, leave it alone.

* **Write your food and your feelings.** By keeping track of what's going into your mouth and what's going on in your life, you gain powerful knowledge you can use to your benefit.

* **Do the best you can with what you know now.** Save perfection for heaven.

Use the USDA Food Pyramid as a guideline:

Grains (bread, cereal, rice, pasta) form the broad base of the pyramid, with a recommended 6 to 11 servings daily. (While you're losing weight, stay at the low end of the recommendation.) One slice of bread, ½ cup pasta or rice, or 1 ounce of cold cereal makes a serving. Whole grains like whole wheat or rye bread, oatmeal, and brown rice are more satisfying and pack more nutrients than refined grains do.

Vegetables, 3 to 5 servings. One cup of leafy greens like spinach or lettuce counts as a serving; so does ½ cup of other vegetables, cooked or raw, or ¾ cup vegetable juice.

Fruit, 2 to 4 servings. A piece of fruit is a serving; so is ¾ cup of fruit juice, but eating whole fruit is more sustaining than drinking juice.

Concentrated proteins (meat, fish, eggs, peanuts, beans, and soy products), 2 to 3 servings. A serving portion is

2 ounces of lean meat (cooked weight), 2 tablespoons peanut butter, or 1 cup (after cooking) of dried beans.

Dairy products or equivalent substitutes, 2 to 3 servings. A serving is 1½ cups milk, yogurt, or calcium-fortified soy or rice beverage; 1½ ounces natural cheese or 2 ounces processed cheese.

Fats, oils, and sugars. At the tip of the pyramid, these are to be used sparingly. In other words, go exceedingly easy on butter, margarine, fatty meats, salad dressings, and desserts other than fresh fruit.

(For more details on the Food Pyramid, visit the Food and Nutrition Information Center's Web site: www.nal usda.gov/fnic/).

These suggestions are too simple and unexciting to be the stuff of mega-selling books and infomercial empires. But they work. If you stick with them, your body will thank you by losing weight and gaining health.

writing prompts

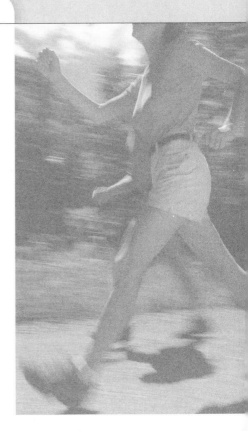

Let these suggestions spur your writing.
Don't feel the need to respond to all of them;
just write about the ones that speak to your heart.

1. You probably know quite a bit about nutrition. Set a timer for five minutes and write as many facts about food as you can in that time. Quick takes—"Fat has twice the calories of protein or carbs"; "Vitamin E is a good antioxidant"—are fine.

2. Be the expert. Write the kind of eating plan that makes the most sense to you. How close does the way you eat now come to this? What can you do to bridge the gap, even a little, today?

3. Where are the holes in your nutritional knowledge? What confuses you? Write your questions. Resolve that during the next seven days you'll get these questions answered. (Consult a registered dietician, or log on to the Web site of the American Dietetic Association, www.eatright.org.)

4. Take a culinary trip down memory lane by writing about the way you ate when you were growing up. What were your favorite foods? Were fresh foods or convenience foods more the norm in your family? How can you eat more healthfully and still satisfy your need for *comfort* or *memory* foods?

5. Put a drop of food coloring in a glass of water. Drink it. You have just ingested truth serum. Now write with rigorous honesty about any foods that you simply cannot eat moderately and forget about. Are these the same foods you believe you can't live without? Are you, just one day at a time, willing to try?

how is my diet?

For one week, keep track of the number of servings you eat of each food group. Don't judge yourself, simply learn about what you are eating. At the end of the week write down your observations, and consider ways to incorporate a more balanced diet into your lifestyle. From time to time, repeat this exercise to continue observing the types of food you are eating.

	MONDAY	TUESDAY	WEDNESDAY	THURSDAY	FRIDAY	SATURDAY	SUNDAY
grains							
vegetables							
fruit							
concentrated proteins							
dairy products or equivalent substitutes							
fats, oils, and sugars							

observations about my week

nourish
and nurture

Food I ate today:

Exercise I did:

Something to care for me:

*More people will die from
hit-or-miss eating than from
hit-and-run driving.*

DUNCAN HINES

nourish
and nurture

Food I ate today:

Exercise I did:

Something to care for me:

Eating is not merely a material pleasure. Eating gives a spectacular joy to life and contributes immensely to good will and happy companionship.

ELSA SCHIAPARELLI

nourish
and nurture

Food I ate today:

Exercise I did:

Something to care for me:

The most prevalent flavor of life is bittersweet.

ANONYMOUS

nourish
and nurture

Food I ate today:

Exercise I did:

Something to care for me:

nourish
and nurture

Food I ate today:

Exercise I did:

Something to care for me:

nourish
and nurture

Food I ate today:

Exercise I did:

Something to care for me:

*There is no love sincerer than
the love of food.*

GEORGE BERNARD SHAW

nourish
and nurture

Food I ate today:

Exercise I did:

Something to care for me:

*The food was stunning,
original, precise, provocative,
and very delicious. These are
the five things we ask of
modern cooking, aren't they?*

JEFFREY STEINGARTEN

Inside us there is a voice of balance that allows us to eat a wide range of foods—for me, the range goes from fine chocolate to roasted vegetables—if we're just easy about it all.

LIZ BROWN

nourish
and nurture

Food I ate today:

Exercise I did:

Something to care for me:

check in

Use this page to help you focus on where you are in the process of achieving body confidence. What are your frustrations? What are your achievements?

chapter **3**

the exercise piece

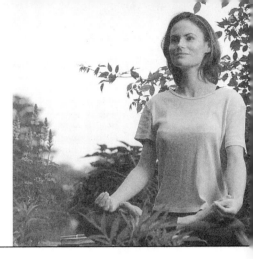

When you've been eating well for a while, you'll feel better about yourself and you'll actually *want* to exercise. Conversely, if you undertake an exercise program—even something as simple as walking half an hour a few days a week—you'll have more energy, greater confidence, and a more positive attitude. It follows that you'll soon want to eat more healthfully, too.

The secret to making exercise part of your life is just that: Make it part of your life, not some alien invader. If, for example, you're a working mom who has to get children to school at eight-thirty and be at the office at nine, signing up for morning swim classes is probably out of the question. A lunch-hour yoga session on Monday and Friday and an after-work Tae-Bo class on Tuesday and Thursday while the kids have soccer would make more sense.

Besides, exercise doesn't always have to be structured. People who are naturally slim tend to be naturally active. They walk to do errands in the neighborhood. They get up to refill their own glass of water. They enjoy energetic hobbies—gardening, sports, dancing.

Not being one of those people myself, I had to look—

and look pretty hard—to find activities I enjoyed. I started with yoga because it didn't seem like exercise. I progressed to city walks, both because I find the changing scene of urban streets endlessly fascinating, and because when I can walk *to* something, that doesn't seem like exercise either. Then I rediscovered the single athletic activity I had excelled at as a youngster: roller-skating. It doesn't seem like exercise because it's so much fun. Writing in your journal can help you discover mobile pursuits you'll like doing. When you find them, you'll no longer have to force yourself to exercise.

Some people prefer aerobic exercise, "slow burn" activities like walking, running, biking, swimming, and step or spinning classes. Others like the feeling of power they get from resistance exercise—rowing, rock climbing, working out with free weights, or using weight machines at a gym. Since both kinds of exercise encourage weight loss, and you need both to be in peak form, experiment with the one you're less fond of and see if you can warm up to it. Adding stretching to your routine will help keep your body young and supple.

Design your life so that exercising is easier than not exercising. See that the activities you choose fit both your schedule and your personality. If you're an extrovert, lone country hikes probably aren't for you. If you're happiest in your own company, I don't recommend a noisy, crowded gym known for its gregarious staff. If you get bored with what you're doing—even just a little—try something different. And if you're over forty or have any condition that requires a doctor's care, get the green light from your health professional before you start exercising.

Yes, physical activity can be good for you. And, yes, it will help you lose weight. In a way, that's too bad. If it were a little bit sinful, we'd probably find it easier to jump in with both feet and simply enjoy the feeling.

writing prompts

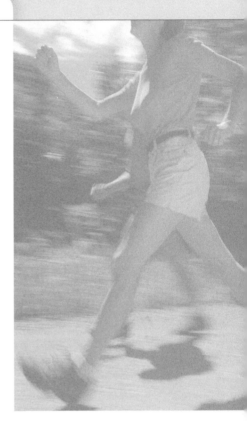

Let these suggestions spur your writing.
Don't feel the need to respond to all of them;
just write about the ones that speak to your heart.

1. Write the highlights of your life story *from your body's point of view.* List some of the peak experiences for your physical self. How much fun has *it* had? Did it get to play enough when you were a child? Does it get to play enough now? How would your physical self like things to be different?

2. Jot down your typical day's routine with the intention of finding places to include more "incidental exercise." Where can you walk to instead of driving? Where can you take the stairs instead of the elevator? How can you become more mobile at home, at the office, on the weekends?

3. Pretend that formal exercise is a person. What kind of relationship do the two of you have? Are you in love? Estranged friends? Mortal enemies? Go to an imaginary relationship counselor. Write the counselor's advice for helping you and exercise become closer and get along better.

4. Make a list of everything active that you truly enjoy. This can include exercise. Sports. Hobbies that take some muscle. Chores that require you to get up and move around, like walking the dog or mowing the lawn. (And of course you can write down sex; this is your private journal.)

5. Prioritize the items in the list you made for prompt 4. "C" items are okay, "B" activities are better, and "A's"

are out of this world. Now figure out how you'll put more of these into your life—the A's especially. If your list is short—or the page is blank—write the activities you *wish* you enjoyed, maybe some that you used to do but think you're too heavy, too old, or too out of shape to do now. Just write them. You may discover something you didn't expect.

6. Revise history. If you have unpleasant memories around physical activity—being made fun of in gym class maybe, or being chosen last for teams—write about one of these experiences. Then rewrite the story the way it *should* have happened. In this version, you got to dance the part of the swan, not hide in the back row. In this rendition, you weren't just chosen to play; you were team captain and hit the winning run.

nourish
and nurture

Food I ate today:

Exercise I did:

Something to care for me:

nourish
and nurture

Food I ate today:

Exercise I did:

Something to care for me:

*In my youth, before I lost any
of my senses, I can remember
that I was all alive, and
inhabited my body with
inexpressible satisfaction.*

HENRY DAVID THOREAU

Wake up and treat your body like it is someone you really care about. Hug yourself. Stretch. Murmur a sweet everything when you look in the mirror. You will feel energized, delighted, and powerful.

DEBORAH SHOUSE

nourish *and nurture*

Food I ate today:

Exercise I did:

Something to care for me:

*It is a happy talent to know
how to play.*

RALPH WALDO EMERSON

nourish
and nurture

Food I ate today:

Exercise I did:

Something to care for me:

nourish
and nurture

Food I ate today:

Exercise I did:

Something to care for me:

nourish *and nurture*

Food I ate today:

Exercise I did:

Something to care for me:

Vitality shows in not only the ability to persist, but in the ability to start over.

F. Scott Fitzgerald

nourish
and nurture

Food I ate today:

Exercise I did:

Something to care for me:

I never met an exercise I liked so instead of working out, I have recess. It's a mind game but it works.

KAREN ROWINSKY,
*COME ALIVE! 50 EASY WAYS TO
HAVE MORE ENERGY NOW*

nourish *and nurture*

Food I ate today:

Exercise I did:

Something to care for me:

I just tired of "living life in the fat lane," so I took the steps to find my sanity.

Jay Mulvaney

check in

Use this page to help you focus on where you are in the process of achieving body confidence. What are your frustrations? What are your achievements?

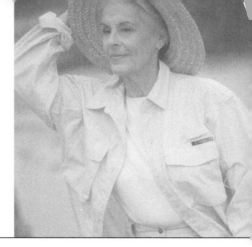

the acceptance edge

So often when we feel down on ourselves, we're really down on our bodies. Living in a culture that is obsessed with appearance, we compare ourselves to models and movie stars, and we chastise ourselves for not measuring up. This will never help us lose weight because it engenders self-loathing, the diametric opposite of body confidence.

Body confidence is accepting ourselves today and allowing ourselves to be better tomorrow. "Better" doesn't mean thin as a rake. It means stronger. Healthier. More self-assured. Eating right and exercising build these qualities. So does deciding every morning—and throughout the day if necessary—that you are as valuable right now as you're ever going to be. Losing weight will not change your innate worth one iota. What it will do is help you have more energy, more choices, and perhaps even more years to enjoy your life.

Hard as it may be to believe if you haven't been thin for a long time, thinness will not by itself make you feel good about who you are. That's an inside job. In fact, if you don't start appreciating yourself now, you'll expect your weight loss to do something it can't possibly accomplish: change what's between your ears.

Because the media is such a ubiquitous force in our society, you may have bought into the cultural party line about body size more than you think. If you're hypercritical of your own body or of other people's, you may be an unwitting advocate of a system that rates people by how little they weigh and how much they own.

This is a dangerous precedent because bodies and situations change all the time. Women get pregnant. Men get sick. One season you may be shopping at exclusive boutiques, another at discount stores. Should any of these exterior circumstances affect how you regard yourself, your weight loss will be on shaky ground. Instead, think well of yourself regardless of your measurements or your demographics. Take care of yourself because you play a vital role in this world and in the lives of those who love you.

Try the following:

* **Make friends who think you're terrific.** Or make *more* friends who think you're terrific. You can never have too many. Sometimes the friends who understand you best are those who have shared similar struggles. For this reason, joining a weight-loss club or organization can provide you not only with useful ideas about eating better and living well, but with a support system of people who know what you've gone through—and who are with you all the way.

* **Treat yourself exceedingly well.** This means eating when you're hungry, resting when you're tired, and saying no when you need to. It means giving yourself the same level of attention and care you give to someone you think is fabulous—your child, for instance. It even includes the occasional indulgence; you deserve the best you can afford. (You probably deserve *better* than you can afford, but we all have to deal with the restrictions

of reality.) Figure out how you can care for yourself in the way to which you'd like to become accustomed. Once you know what you want, you're more likely to come up with the wherewithal for at least some of it.

* **Take quiet time just for you.** Having quiet time every day will help you lose weight and develop enough serenity that you'll be less likely to regain it. Sitting each day for meditation, prayer, journal writing, or a blend of these, will help you learn to stay still. This skill is transferable; you can use it to calm yourself, center yourself, and stay out of the kitchen when you feel a hankering for some food you don't need. Quiet time also gives you a way to frame your day, starting it with peacefulness and ending it with gratitude.

In the most basic sense, self-acceptance is being in your own corner. It's allowing yourself to be human and have human failings, while at the same time appreciating the unique array of attributes that makes you the only person like you who has ever lived. It's making peace with who you are, thighs and all, so you're free to relish every delicious morsel of every day you've got.

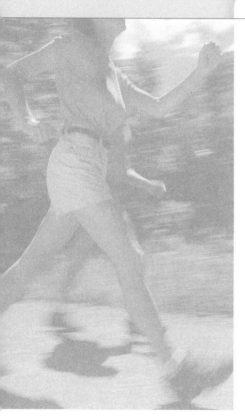

writing prompts

Let these suggestions spur your writing.
Don't feel the need to respond to all of them;
just write about the ones that speak to your heart.

1. Describe your concept of the ideal body type for some-
    one of your age and gender. Then write where this
    notion came from—parents, spouse, friends, TV, maga-
    zines? Is achieving this look even possible for you, and
    if it is, could you maintain it without constant upkeep?
    If not, can you amend your ideal to one that is realistic
    for you?

2. List the names of twenty people you know personally
    who look beautiful or handsome to you. How many of
    them look quite different from the cultural ideal of
    attractiveness? What are the qualities that make these
    men and women appealing?

3. Do a reality check. What do you expect to gain from
    losing weight? How do you think it will change your
    life? Are your expectations realistic or are you anticipat-
    ing more than simply a smaller body size can deliver?

4. List adjectives that describe overweight people as a
    group, then read what you've written. Are these words
    complimentary, critical, or a mixture? If those same
    words described a racial or ethnic group, would you say
    they were written by a fair-minded person or a preju-
    diced one? If the latter, what can you do to neutralize
    your judgments?

5. Make a list of ways you would like to nurture yourself that you aren't doing now. Of this list, pick the three you want to do most. Why aren't you enjoying these now? If it's a financial consideration, can you find this kind of nurturing at an affordable price, or can you rearrange your budget to allow for it, at least every once in a while? If you're putting off this delight for some other reason, what are you waiting for?

how can i better accept myself?

Write a letter to yourself describing the steps you need to take to better accept yourself. Pretend you are your own best friend and give encouraging advice about achieving these steps. If you would like, photocopy the letter and ask someone to send it to you in six months. At that time, ask yourself how well you are following your own advice.

Dear _____ ,

Your friend,

Where there is great love,
there are always miracles.

WILLA CATHER

nourish
and nurture

Food I ate today:

Exercise I did:

Something to care for me:

There is a fountain of youth—it is your mind, your talents, the creativity you bring to your life.

SOPHIA LOREN

nourish
and nurture

Food I ate today:

Exercise I did:

Something to care for me:

*Being radiantly healthy,
living fully, and celebrating
life starts with celebrating
ourselves. Whether we
succeed or fail, enjoy our lives
or struggle, depends largely
on our self-image.*

SUSAN SMITH JONES,
CHOOSE TO LIVE PEACEFULLY

nourish *and nurture*

Food I ate today:

Exercise I did:

Something to care for me:

nourish
and nurture

Food I ate today:

Exercise I did:

Something to care for me:

nourish *and nurture*

Food I ate today:

Exercise I did:

Something to care for me:

Row the boat. Let God steer.

ANONYMOUS

nourish *and nurture*

Food I ate today:

Exercise I did:

Something to care for me:

*Before you crawl (or jump)
out of bed in the morning,
stay put and silently say good
morning to the new day. Or
sleep an extra five minutes.
That's peaceful, too.*

LESLIE LEVINE,
ICE CREAM FOR BREAKFAST

If you are irritated by every rub, how will your mirror be polished?

RUMI

nourish *and nurture*

Food I ate today:

Exercise I did:

Something to care for me:

check in

Use this page to help you focus on where you are in the process of achieving body confidence. What are your frustrations? What are your achievements?

chapter 5

living thin

I recently went to a movie with my husband, William, who has never had a weight problem. He had gone all day without eating, so we were in the concession line to get him a snack. "Maybe I'll have a cookie," he mused. "I wonder what kinds those are."

I looked at the case and said, "Peanut butter, oatmeal-raisin, and chocolate chip."

"You can tell that by looking? Then what are those?" he wanted to know, pointing at the muffins.

"Banana-walnut, cranberry-orange, and cinnamon-apple."

"That's amazing. It's too bad there isn't a quiz show you could go on: 'Name That Pastry.'"

We laughed, but I had a sobering revelation at the same time: Even though I have been thin for the better part of two decades, and even though I eat normally and healthfully today with little thought to the matter, my relationship with food will always be different from William's. Although I no longer eat sweets with wild abandon, I will always be able to identify them in a lineup.

For any of us with a history of overeating, the possibility of going back to the old ways is always there. We don't have to be afraid of this—fear is counterproductive—but we do need to be aware of it.

If you overate as a response to uncomfortable emotional states—sadness, rejection, loneliness, anger—your brain's neural pathways are programmed to take the familiar route of "I feel sad; I should eat" or "I feel angry; I should eat." These patterns don't disappear overnight, and even when you think they're gone for good, they sometimes resurface. You don't have to act on them, though. Draw on the tools that helped you change in the first place. Call a friend who understands. Write out your feelings. Sit out the urge, and it *will* go away.

Do not let appearances mislead you. You're the same person at 150 pounds as you were at 180. You've developed new habits and you have accomplished something to be proud of, but it takes much longer to change deeply ingrained mental/emotional responses than it does to lose 30 pounds. Because the thinner person looking back at you from the mirror could still succumb to overeating, realize that you must continue to make the practices that led to your weight loss part of your life for the duration.

If you think about it, losing weight—even losing it slowly, which is of course the best way—does not take a lot of time. Depending on the amount of weight you want to release, it may take six weeks, six months, or twice that long. The maintenance period, however, is the rest of your life.

Realize this fact from the outset and plan accordingly. If you go on a weight-loss diet that you expect to follow up with a weight-maintenance diet, you'll be on a diet all your life. That is certainly not appealing and probably not even possible. Instead, change your lifestyle from the very start to one that supports normal weight over the long haul. Eat well. Exercise as if you actually wanted to. Surround yourself with supportive people and stay in contact with them. Fill the pages of this book, and keep on writing.

You may not want to write your food forever, but knowing how to do it means you can draw on this technique whenever you're feeling shaky, or if you're in a new situation and want a little extra help. And life journaling, writing about your day and your feelings, may well become a lifelong practice. The key to keeping weight off is to know yourself so well that you can see a return to old patterns coming before it moves in and does damage. Journal writing is unparalleled in its ability to keep you aware of what is going on in your psyche.

To continue the journaling process, you might want to buy another journal in this series, or you can simply get yourself a spiral notebook and reuse the *Body Confident* prompts you wrote about weeks or months before. Because you're a growing, changing individual, the prompts will mean something different every time you address them. You might also go back and pick up the ones you skipped this time through. Your writing will keep you grounded and secure. In time you'll realize that you're not just confident about your body, you're thrilled about your life.

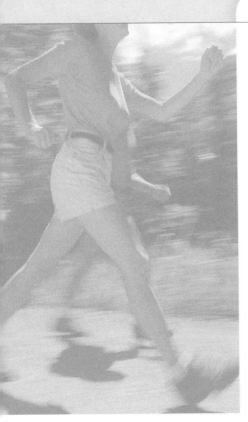

writing prompts

Let these suggestions spur your writing.
Don't feel the need to respond to all of them;
just write about the ones that speak to your heart.

1. For a few minutes, be one of those people who says, "I've got some good news—and some bad news." First write about what is "bad"—difficult, discouraging—about having to pay attention to eating well and exercising regularly, even after you've lost weight. Then come up with a positive spin and write the good news.

2. Think about how difficult it must have been for people 500 years ago to defy what their eyes told them and accept that the earth wasn't flat. You have the same challenge in coming to accept that, even as a slender person, you will still need to employ some vigilance. Write about what it's like (or what it will be like) to be a thin person with a fat history.

3. A lot of people don't pay much attention to the clothes they wear until they've lost weight. Start enjoying your fashionable side *now* by validating what you like today. Answer the following questions in your journal:

    * **What are my favorites**—colors, styles, stores, designers, brands?

    * **What's my style**—traditional, casual, romantic, bohemian, exotic, alluring, artistic, or some combination?

    * **What do I most enjoy wearing now?** What might I want to wear when I've lost half the weight I plan to lose? And when I've lost all of it?

4. Imagine that you're a lifestyle consultant, and a client (in this case, yourself) has asked you to design a comprehensive lifestyle plan for living well, staying thin, and having a strong shot at making your dreams come true. Devise this plan and write it up. Refer to it in the weeks and months ahead. Make revisions when they're necessary.

how am i feeling?

Enlarge your awareness about emotional eating. Write down an emotional state in column 1, a food you might turn to in this state in column 2, and an inedible alternative in column 3. The next time you feel that emotion, check your list for a healthy way to respond to your mood.

sample

EMOTION	MY OLD FOOD RESPONSE	MY NEW HEALTHY RESPONSE
Anger	Chips	Go for a speed walk
Jealousy	Chocolate	Write about it
Elation	Ice cream	Do a short meditation

your turn

EMOTION	MY OLD FOOD RESPONSE	MY NEW HEALTHY RESPONSE

Big shots are only little shots
who keep shooting.

CHRISTOPHER MORLEY

nourish
and nurture

Food I ate today:

Exercise I did:

Something to care for me:

nourish
and nurture

Food I ate today:

Exercise I did:

Something to care for me:

nourish
and nurture

Food I ate today:

Exercise I did:

Something to care for me:

There is no failure except in no longer trying. There is no defeat except from within, no really insurmountable barrier save our own inherent weakness of purpose.

KIN HUBBARD

nourish
and nurture

Food I ate today:

Exercise I did:

Something to care for me:

If a man wants to be sure of his road, he must close his eyes and walk in the dark.

SAINT JOHN OF THE CROSS

Don't smoke too much, drink too much, eat too much, or work too much. We are all on the road to the grave—but there's no reason to be in the passing lane.

ROBERT ORBEN

nourish
and nurture

Food I ate today:

Exercise I did:

Something to care for me:

nourish
and nurture

Food I ate today:

Exercise I did:

Something to care for me:

Have no fear of perfection.
You'll never reach it.

SALVADOR DALI

It's always too early to quit.

NORMAN VINCENT PEALE

nourish *and nurture*

Food I ate today:

Exercise I did:

Something to care for me:

check in

Use this page to help you focus on where you are in the process of achieving body confidence. What are your frustrations? What are your achievements?

for further reading

Love Yourself Thin: The Revolutionary Spiritual Approach to Weight Loss, Victoria Moran (Signet, 1999).

Overcoming Overeating, Jane R. Hirschmann, Carol H. Munter, and C. Peter Herman (Fawcett, 1998).

The Me I Knew I Could Be: One Woman's Journey from 292 Pounds to Peace, Happiness, and Healthy Living, Crystal Phillips (St. Martin's Press, 2001).

The 7 Secrets of Slim People, Vikki Hansen, M.S.W., and Shawn Goodman (Hay House, 1997; HarperPaperbacks, 1999).

Take It Off and Keep It Off: Based on the Successful Methods of Overeaters Anonymous, Anonymous (NTC/Contemporary, 1989).

Thin for Life: 10 Keys to Success from People Who Have Lost Weight and Kept It Off, Anne M. Fletcher, M.S., R.D. (Chapters Publishing, Ltd., 1994).

Turn Off the Fat Genes: The Revolutionary Guide to Taking Charge of the Genes that Control Your Weight, Neal D. Barnard, M.D. (Harmony Books, 2001).

When You Eat at the Refrigerator, Pull Up a Chair: 50 Ways to Feel Thin, Gorgeous, and Happy (When You Feel Anything But), Geneen Roth (Hyperion, 1999).